SLEEP

Discover How to Fall Asleep More Easily

Kalykakis Georgios

Kalykakis Georgios

Sleep: Discover How to Fall Asleep More Easily

information is without contract or any type of guarantee assurance. The trademarks that are used are without any consent, and the publication of the trademark is without permission or backing by the trademark owner. All trademarks and brands within this book are for clarifying purposes only and are the owned by the owners themselves, not affiliated with this document.

Kalykakis Georgios

Table of Contents

Introduction

Many people have problems falling asleep and staying asleep. Insomnia and sleep deprivation can cause people to act differently than they normally would. Insomnia and sleep deprivation can also affect productivity and cause health problems. If you are experiencing sleep issues, the information in this book will make you happier, healthier and more productive in no time. You'll learn why we need sleep, and how to achieve the sleep that's currently eluding you.

Chapter 1: Sleep Is Crucial

Sleep plays a very crucial role in ensuring you stay in good health. Getting enough of it at the right time will protect your mental and physical health. It will also provide you with a better quality of life.

The way a person feels during their waking hours depends on what happens during their sleeping hours. During sleep, the body will work to support healthy brain function and maintain physical health. Children and teenagers need enough sleep in order to support healthy growth and good development. Infants may need more than 16 hours of sleep daily, whereas preschool children will need to nap. Young children sleep more in the early evening, while teenagers tend to sleep more during the morning.

Deep sleep in growing children will trigger the release of the hormone that helps promote growth, boost muscle mass, and help repair cells and tissue. Sleep also helps teenagers transition through puberty and promotes fertility. Without enough sleep children and teenagers can have problems getting along with their peers, become impulsive or angry, and suffer from mood swings, depression, stress, and a lack of motivation. They may also have issues paying attention and their grades will begin to suffer. One particular study of teenagers showed that with every hour of lost sleep, the odds of being overweight also increased.

Damage from lack of sleep can happen instantly like a car wreck, or it can harm a person over time. When a person continuously does not get enough sleep, potential chronic health issues aren't the only problem. Lack of sleep can also affect how a person reacts, thinks, learns, works, and even how they get along with other people.

There are many people that do not recognize the terrible toll that not sleeping will take on their mental and cognitive health. Many of those people think that sleep is nothing more than a luxury. They understand that they will feel better with a full night's sleep, and then worse when they do not. However, sleep will actually improve memory, learning, as well as insight.

Good Brain Function and Emotional Health

Sleep helps the brainwork efficiently. While a person sleeps at night, the brain is preparing for the following day. It is creating new pathways to help you learn, as well as offering ways to remember information. Studies have shown that having a good night's sleep will improve a person's learning and problem-solving abilities: whether it's learning to play the piano or learning math, trying to perfect a golf swing or learning how to drive. Getting regular sleep will also help a person to pay closer attention, make wiser decisions, and enhance their creativity.

Studies have shown that lack of sleep will alter activity in parts of the brain. If a person is sleep deprived, they may have a hard time making decisions, controlling their emotions and behavior, solving problems, and coping. Sleep deprivation has also been linked to risk taking, depression, and even suicide.

Sleep and Physical Health

Sleep plays a large role in a person's physical health. For example, sleep helps the body heal and repair the heart, along with the blood vessels. Ongoing lack of sleep is directly linked to increased heart disease, high blood pressure, kidney disease, stroke, diabetes, and obesity.

Sleep also balances the body's hormones, causing a person to feel hungry or full. When a person does not get enough sleep the body's level of ghrelin - the hormone that makes you hungry - increases, while Leptin - the hormone that makes you feel full - decreases. A decrease in Leptin will cause a person to overeat and gain weight. By getting enough sleep, a person will eat less and lose the weight they initially gained due to lack of sleep.

Sleep also affects how the body reacts to insulin. Insulin is the hormone that controls the body's blood glucose level. Lack of sleep will result in a higher blood glucose level, thereby increasing the risk of developing diabetes.

The immune system also relies on sleep in order to stay healthy. This specific system defends the body against harmful and foreign substances. Ongoing sleep issues will change the way the immune system responds. For example, if a person does not get enough sleep, they will have issues fighting common illnesses and infections.

Safety and Daytime Performance

Getting enough sleep during at the right times will help a person function well throughout the day. Those who do not get enough sleep normally take longer to finish assigned tasks, react more slowly, and may make more mistakes than they normally would. After many nights of lack of sleep, even if it is just a couple hours each night, the ability to function will suffer and the effects are as if the person had not slept for one or two days.

Sleep deficiency can also lead to microsleep. Microsleep are quick moments of sleep that can happen when a person is normally awake. A person cannot control microsleep, and they may not be aware of it happening. For example, a person who drives to work may not remember having done so. Microsleep affects how a person functions. If someone is listening to a lesson or lecture, they may miss some of the information or feel as though they do not understand the points. In reality, they may have just slept through parts of it and are not aware they did so.

Some people aren't aware of the risks of not getting enough sleep. They may not even realize they aren't sleeping enough and believe they are still able to function efficiently. A great example is a sleepy driver. Studies have shown lack of sleep impairs driving ability as much as - and in some cases even more than - drinking and driving. It is estimated that sleep-deprived drivers causes approximately 100,000 accidents every year, resulting in 1,500 deaths per year.

Those who work in the healthcare industry, pilots, mechanics, and even assembly line staff, run the risk of causing harm not only to themselves but others if they don't get enough sleep. Lack of sleep has played a very large role in many human errors that are linked to large tragic accidents like nuclear reactor meltdowns, aviation wrecks, and the grounding of large ships.

What Makes a Person Sleep?

There are many different factors that play a role in preparing the body to fall asleep and wake up. Everyone has an internal clock that controls this process. The internal clock is on a 24-hour repetitive rhythm. There are two processes that interact in order to control the rhythm. The first process is a pressure to fall asleep that builds with each hour during waking hours. This is a drive for sleep that will reach a peak in the evening hours when most people fall asleep.

Sleep: Discover How to Fall Asleep More Easily

A compound by the name of Adenosine seems to be one of the factors linked to the need for sleep. While a person is awake, the level of Adenosine in the brain will continue to increase. This will signal a shift towards sleeping. While a person sleeps, their body will break down the Adenosine.

The second process involves the internal clock. The clock is actually in sync with the cues in the surrounding environment. Darkness, light, and other cues will help the body determine when it feels awake and when it feels tired. For example, light will signal a special area in the brain that tells the body it is daytime. The area of the brain will help align the clock with a certain period of the day and night.

The body will release the chemicals in a rhythm, which the clock controls. When night comes, the body will release the hormone melatonin. Melatonin signals to the body that it is time to get ready for sleep and it will help you feel tired. The quantity of melatonin in the bloodstream will peak as the evening continues. Researchers believe this peak is a very important factor in preparing the body for sleep.

Being exposed to a bright artificial light late at night will disrupt the internal clock, making it difficult to fall asleep. Bright artificial lights can be found in televisions, computer screens or numbers on some alarm clocks.

As the sun comes up, the body releases cortisol. This hormone prepares the body to wake up. The rhythm and timing of a person's internal clock changes as they age. Teenagers end up falling asleep later than younger children and some adults because the melatonin being released peaks later in the cycle. As a result, it is natural for teenagers to want to go to sleep later at night and sleep in in the morning.

The patterns and types of sleep will also change, as people get older. For example, a newborn will spend more time in REM sleep. Non-REM sleep will peak in the early stages of childhood, drop after puberty, and continue to decrease as people age.

Non-REM Sleep

Three phrases happen during non-REM sleep. Each of the stages will last from five minutes up to fifteen minutes. You will go through all of the phases before you actually reach REM sleep.

- *Stage 1*: This is where the eyes are closed; however, it is very easy to wake up. This phase can last from five minutes up to ten minutes
- *Stage 2*: This is a light sleep. The heart rate will slow and the body temperature will drop. He body is getting itself ready to sleep.
- *Stage 3*: This is a stage where deep sleep happens. It is much harder to wake during this stage. If this person were woken suddenly they would be disoriented. During this stage, the body grows and repairs tissues, builds muscle and bone, and even strengthens the body's immune system. As a person gets older, they sleep more lightly, and in turn gets less deep sleep.

REM Sleep

Typically, REM sleep will happen about 90 minutes after a person falls asleep. The first period normally lasts for 10 minutes. Each of the later stages will get longer, and then the final one will only last about an hour. The heart rate and breathing will quicken. People will have intense dreams during their REM sleep. This is because the brain is more active.

Chapter 2: Sleep Deficiency and Deprivation

Sleep deprivation occurs when a person suffers from one or more of the following:

- Does not get enough sleep.
- Sleeps during the wrong times of the day.
- Does not sleep very well or falls asleep at different times than the body needs.
- Has a sleep disorder, which prevents them from sleeping or causes bad sleep.

To understand sleep deficiency, it's important to first understand how sleep actually works and why it is so important. The two types of sleep are REM (rapid eye movement) and non-REM. Non-REM sleep is commonly called deep sleep or slow wave sleep. Dreaming happens during REM sleep. Typically, non-REM and REM sleep happen in a pattern of three to five cycles every night.

The ability to function and feel good while you are awake depends on whether you are getting enough of both REM and Non-REM sleep and whether you are sleeping when the body is ready to sleep.

The body has an internal clock called the body clock. It controls when a person wakes up and goes to sleep. Typically, it follows a 24-hour rhythm called the circadian rhythm. The rhythm will affect every tissue, cell, and organ and how they function. If a person does not get enough sleep or is sleeping at different times, they will find it much harder to judge the emotions of others, including their reactions. It will also make them feel cranky, frustrated, or even worried in social situations.

A health survey conducted by the Centers for Disease Control and Prevention revealed that between seven and 19 percent of adults in the United States reported they weren't getting enough sleep.

Almost 40 percent of adults reported falling asleep through the day without actually meaning to at least once during the month. And an estimated 50 to 70 million people have chronic sleep disorders. Sleep deprivation has been directly linked to chronic health issues, including kidney disease, heart disease, high blood pressure, stroke, diabetes, obesity and depression.

Signs of Sleeping Problems

Sleep issues can cause a person to feel extremely tired through the day. A person may not feel very refreshed or alert when they wake up if they are suffering from a sleep disorder.

How sleepy a person feels during the day can help determine if they are having issues. A person has sleep issues if they experience any of the following:

- Falling asleep while watching television.
- Falling asleep while reading a book.
- Falling asleep while riding inside of a car for an hour.
- Falling asleep while sitting and speaking with someone.
- Falling asleep after lunch.
- Falling asleep while in traffic.

If you find that you have issues sleeping, then you may have a sleeping disorder. Here are the sleeping disorders with the signs. If you find that you have signs that match any of these, then you will need to speak with a doctor.

- *Insomnia*: Those with insomnia have a hard time falling asleep. They will wake up during the night and then have issues falling back to sleep. They will have "racing" thoughts while they are trying to fall asleep.
- *Restless Leg Syndrome*: Those with restless leg syndrome will experience a crawling sensation in the legs. They may even have involuntary leg jerks once they lay down to try to sleep. Leg cramps will also happen during sleep and will keep the person up.
- *Sleep Apnea*: Those with sleep apnea will snore. They will also stop breathing while they are sleeping. These people will also have high blood pressure. Sleep apnea also causes people to feel tired even after a night of sleeping.

There are things that can cause sleep disorders like insomnia.

- Having a brain injury.
- Schedules that will keep you awake and not allow you to sleep.
- Taking drugs that mimic neurotransmitters like caffeine or cocaine.
- There are unusual circumstances that can also be an issue. Circumstances can be hunger, severe pain, high carbon dioxide levels, inner ear issues, and zero gravity.

Substances that Cause Sleep Disorders

- *Caffeine*: This is the mostly used stimulant. It blocks adenosine with makes a person sleepy. People use caffeine in order to stay awake and even increase alertness. However, it will make it very hard to fall asleep during the night.
- *Nicotine*: This is another stimulant. It will affect those who need to go to sleep and those who smoke often will

experience withdrawal symptoms very quickly. They will also wake up earlier than normal due to withdrawals too.

- *Recreational Drugs and Prescription Medications*: These two types of drugs, legal or not, will also keep a person from sleeping normally.

Light and Sleeplessness

Light is a very huge reason why people stay awake and not get enough sleep. Light keeps people alert. Light is even utilized to keep pilots awake in the Air Force. Light therapy is utilized for the treatment of circadian disorders. An over abundance of light will prevent sleep and cause a person to wake up earlier than they are supposed too.

The proliferation of the electronic devices has raised problems for those that are prone to light disruption. Computer screens, televisions, and other devices make it hard for a person to sleep. Those who research this issue refer to it as EECD, meaning electronic entertainment and communication devices.

Other Types of Disruptors

The relationship with sleep and pain is a complicated one. It depends a bit on the source of the person's pain, the location in their body, and the severity. Pain will make it difficult to sleep; however, it will also encourage the person's brain to stay asleep since the body needs to heal itself. For the traumatic pain that keeps a person awake, the person may need to take over the counter pain medicine or prescription pain management medicine in order to relieve the pain so they are able to sleep.

Exercise and Sleep

Exercise is one of the things that will come in different forms, which will have different effects on a person's sleep quality, as well as quantity.

- Daytime Exercising: This is great for a person's sleep.
- Evening Exercising: If it is done after work, yet before dinner it is great for sleep.
- Nighttime Exercising: This will keep you awake and make it very hard to go to sleep.

Although those are generalization, some people will have no issue with nighttime exercising. This is the same way that some people have no issue with drinking caffeine before bed. Daytime exercising can also be the opposite for somewhere it is just too much stimulus for them to go to bed during the nighttime hours.

Chapter 3: How Much Sleep Is Needed?

It is very important that people get the necessary amount of sleep. How much sleep a person needs changes as they age and varies from person to person. The table shows how much sleep is recommended based on a person's age.

AGE	AMOUNT OF SLEEP
Newborns	14 - 17 Hours
4 to 11 Months	12 - 15 Hours
Toddlers 1 - 2 Years	11 - 14 Hours
Preschool Age 3 - 5 Years	10 - 13 Hours
School Age 6 - 13 Years	9 - 11 Hours
Teenage 14 - 17 Years	7 - 9 Hours
Young Adult 18 - 25 Years	7 - 9 Hours
Adults 26 - 64 Years	7 - 9 Hours
Older Adults 65 Years and Older	7 - 8 Hours

It is important to note that young children need a lot of sleep. This is typically broken up into bedtime and then a nap in the middle of the day. This will ensure that they get the necessary energy to get through the day.

Sleep: Discover How to Fall Asleep More Easily

If a person loses sleep on a regular basis or chooses to sleep less, the sleep loss adds up. The total amount of sleep lost is called sleep debt. For example, if a person loses two hours of sleep every night, they will have a sleep debt of about 14 hours after just one week. There are some people who nap in order to deal with the sleepiness. Naps actually provide a short-term boost, making a person more alert and increasing activity. However, just napping does not provide all the other benefits that come from a night's sleep. Thus, if a person cannot make up for the lost sleep they will still be in sleep debt.

There are some people who sleep more during their days off work. They will also go to bed later and get up later. Sleeping more on days off may be a sign that a person is not getting enough sleep. Although extra sleep on days off may help a person feel better, it may also upset the body's sleep-wake balance. Having a bad sleep habit and long-term loss of sleep will affect a person's health. If you're worried about getting enough sleep, try keeping a sleep diary for a couple weeks. If you decide you need a sleep diary, write down the amount of sleep that you get every night. You will also need to write down how alert you feel, as well as how rested you feel every morning. You also need to record how sleepy you feel throughout the day. Show the records to your doctor and discuss how to improve your sleeping habits.

It is important to sleep when your body needs to. Even if you're getting enough sleep, you may still be out of sync with your internal body clock. People who may be out of sync include mothers of small children, shift workers, or those who get interrupted routinely during sleep. If you have a job or daily routine that limits your ability to get the right amount of sleep, discuss the problem with your doctor.

Chapter 4: Falling Asleep More Easily and Faster: Adults

Bad sleep is nothing to shrug off. It will take a toll on your body and affect your job performance, sex life, and your overall health. Follow these steps to ensure that you get enough sleep.

- *Get rid of annoying sounds*. From snoring spouses to delivery trucks beeping, whatever is keeping you awake needs to be tuned out. Relaxing soundtracks are a great way to block out the noise. You can even buy headphones that can be worn comfortably during while you sleep.
- *Prepare your body for sleep*. A progressive technique utilized by Catherine Daley, MD, the director of the Institute of Naturopathic Sleep Medicine in Seattle, suggests curling your toes very tightly for seven seconds. Relax and then repeat the process through each of your muscle groups, working up to your neck.
- *Take some notes*. Daily routines will affect how you sleep at night. Keeping a sleep log will help you make connections as to why you're sleeping well. Each day, record how much caffeine you drink, when you drink it, and how much you exercise. You will need to keep track of what you are eating, when time you go to bed, and what time you wake up. Then total the amount of your sleep time.
- *Keep yourself cool*. People end up dozing off a lot easier and sleep much better when the room is cooler. Set the thermostat to approximately 65 degrees Fahrenheit or even lower. If you get premenopausal sweats or even hot flashes remove the covers, use a cooling mattress pad, moisture wicking sheets, or wear cotton pajamas.

- *Relax the right way*. Instead of going over the daily events once you get into bed, try writing about important things two hours before you go to bed. This will get your mind off things and stop your thoughts racing once you go to bed. Right before bedtime, use relaxing imagery to picture a tranquil scene, like a day at the park or the beach. Over time, your new routine will teach your brain to rest.

Falling Asleep More Easily and Faster: Teenagers

Sleep deprivation among teenagers is a big issue, especially for those with busy days. School, jobs, sports, and other active events are not places where they should be feeling tired. Here are ways for teenagers to get more and better sleep.

- Plan in advance:
  - Do not eat before bedtime. Food creates more energy and will activate the muscles in the stomach, keeping teens up at night. If a teenager plans on going to sleep before 11 p.m. don't let them eat anything after 9:30 p.m. If they are extremely hungry, a small snack is recommended.
  - Take a hot shower a couple of hours before bedtime. It is also important to blow-dry your hair. Wet hair can cause illness or make it harder to fall asleep.
  - Stop watching television and using computers before going to bed. Studies show screen time will keep a person from falling asleep if it is an hour before bedtime.
  - Before falling asleep, do something relaxing. Instead of strenuous activities like exercising,

talk with friends or family members, read, or write in a journal.

- ○ Get dressed for bed. If it's very cold, wear a robe and some slippers. Stay warm, yet comfortable.
- ○ Find the right things before bedtime. If it's cold, make sure you have enough blankets. If it's warm, wear appropriate pajamas and make sure you have a fan.
- ○ You will need to floss and brush your teeth, drink some water, wash and dry your face, brush your hair and use the bathroom. Doing so will help you feel clean and comfortable.
- ○ Before going to bed, write down anything that you need to do tomorrow so that you can rest better.

Get the mind ready:

- ○ Adjust your lighting. Some people need darkness to sleep while others need dim light. Having the right amount of light is important to be comfortable enough to fall asleep.
- ○ Make sure that you are comfortable in the bed. Find a comfortable, warm, to make you feel calm.
- ○ Make sure to set the alarm clock to the right volume and for the specified time that you need to wake up.
- ○ Read a bit of a book or do something that does not cause noise. You can even make up a story in your mind.
- ○ Make a playlist of soft songs or some soothing sounds to help you fall asleep more easily. Try listening to an audio book or talk radio.

What to do once the lights are out:

- ○ Do not worry about how much sleep you are going to get. Doing so will make you less likely to fall asleep. Distract yourself from thinking.

- Once you are comfortable, just close your eyes. Replay the day back in your head and then think of what you did or didn't do. Think about what you accomplished.
- Make sure that you completely relax, and then tell yourself that you will fall asleep. Do not think too much. If something comes into your mind, just push it away.

Other Tips for Falling Asleep

- Shut your eyes and think about something peaceful.
- Concentrate on your breathing. Because it is involuntary, you will forget about it and fall asleep.
- Imagine yourself in a spot that makes you feel peaceful and calm, like a grassy meadow, empty room, or a pond.
- Keep your bedtime and waking time consistent. Establishing a consistent routine will help you get a normal amount of sleep.
- Keep the room cooler.
- Do not eat before bed.
- Listen to relaxing music with your eyes closed as you lay down.
- Use the bathroom before you go to bed.
- Keep a bottle of water by the bed just in case you wake up. Walking to get water will wake you up more and make it harder to go back to sleep.
- Use a sleeping mask to make it darker.
- If you find that you need the television on, make sure the volume is not too high and the show is not too interesting to keep you awake.
- Sleep with a pet on the bed if it makes you feel safer and more secure.
- Sleep with a big stuffed animal if it will help you feel more secure.

- Try deep breathing exercises with your eyes closed.
- Do not think about important issues. Make your thoughts light.
- Do not think of anything bad from that day or the day before.
- Do not take any sleep medication. It will cause restlessness and unhealthy sleeping patterns.
- Do not eat sugar before bed.
- Drink a warm cup of tea.
- Drink a warm cup of milk.
- Take a hot shower a couple of hours before bed, but go to bed with dry hair.
- Brush your teeth and wash your face.

Conclusion

As you have read, it is crucial to make sure you get enough sleep. Some of the tips will work for you, while others may not. Everyone is different. Try what you think will work. If it doesn't, move on to the next tip. Once you find what works for you, make it a routine. Your body will then take this routine as a cue to get ready to sleep. Keep in mind that you will also need to seek help from a doctor if nothing seems to improve your sleeping patterns. It can be a sign of an underlying medical issue. And remember, just because you take a nap does not mean that you are meeting the sleep quota that you need for your age group.

Book Description:
You are able to end your fatigue and your sleepless nights with the help of this book. Those who read this book will learn easy tips in order to solve the sleeping issues. Just imagine how getting a good night's sleep will feel. You will finally get to enjoy life once again and feel fully energized. The sleeping secrets in this book will give you a new way to approach bedtime. From sleep deprivation to insomnia, this book will offer you information on how to sleep, why you sleep, and so much more. If you answer yes to any of these questions, then this book is for you:

- You wake up exhausted after a full night's sleep.
- You are having issues sleeping, even when you feel tired.
- You take more than twenty minutes in order to fall asleep or even back to sleep once you have woke up.
- You are taking pills in order to sleep.
- You feel depressed or moody.

- You snore or have sleep apnea.
- Your sex life is suffering from a lack of energy or desire.

This book offers different ways for you to fall asleep and turn your life around. Sleep is needed for your physical and your mental health. In this book is information for your body to get back on track where is should be.

www.ingramcontent.com/pod-product-compliance
Lightning Source LLC
Chambersburg PA
CBHW061953280526
45787CB00004B/1837